Type 1 Diabetes

and

Babysitting

A Parent's Toolkit

Includes Pull-Out Pages for Babysitters

by

Stacey Smith-Bradfield and Dayna Frei

Science Horse Productions LLC
P.O. Box 38879
Colorado Springs, CO 80937
www.sciencehorseproductions.com

ISBN 978-0-615-86345-0

All images in this book are copyrighted by their respective authors.

NovoLog®, Levemir® and FlexPen® are registered trademarks of Novo Nordisk A/S. Novo Nordisk A/S manufactures the GlucaGen HypoKit. Humalog® and Humalog® KwikPen™ are registered trademarks of Eli Lilly and Company. Lantus® and Apidra® are registered trademarks of sanofi-aventis U.S. LLC . The glucagon design is a trademark of Eli Lilly and Company. Eli Lilly and Company manufactures the Glucagon Emergency Rescue Kit. CalorieKing™ is a registered trademark of CalorieKing Wellness Solutions, Inc.

Ordering Information: Quantity sales. Special discounts are available on quantity purchases by corporations, associations, and others. For details, contact the authors at the address above.

Printed in the United States of America

This book is dedicated to

Quincy Bradfield and Hannah Frei,

our inspiration.

Table of Contents

Medical Disclaimer

This book is designed to provide you with information about diabetes management. It is sold with the understanding that the authors and publisher are not engaged in rendering medical advice. This book is not intended to provide a complete or exhaustive treatment of this subject; nor is it a substitute for advice from your child's physician or diabetes care provider, who know your child best.

All efforts were made to ensure the accuracy of information contained in this publication as of the date of writing. The authors and publisher expressly disclaim any responsibility for any adverse effects arising from the use or application of the information contained herein. While the parties believe that the contents of this application are accurate, a licensed medical practitioner should be consulted in the event that medical advice is desired. The information contained in this book does not constitute a recommendation or endorsement with respect to any company or product.

Introduction For Parents

As parents of children with diabetes, we understand the mix of emotions that comes with leaving your children in the care of someone other than yourself. After all, no one knows your child better than you! With this guide, we hope to give you as a parent some peace of mind through the critical information needed to manage your child's diabetes. We have laid out the information in a simple manner that can be easily understood and referenced, helping you educate those caring for your child such as a babysitter, grandparent or another parent.

This guide is a roadmap of your child's care. It will help guide and prepare the sitter or other adult in the typical situations that might arise with diabetes while you are away. Because children are individuals, they have different needs for their diabetes (and those needs can change all the time). We have provided this workbook for you to fill out about YOUR child. All the critical information needed is in one place, in one book.

In this book you will have different signs. Information in *ITALICS* indicate instructions specifically for parents. The pen indicates places for the parent to fill in. We suggest using a pencil, keeping in mind that information about your child is continually changing. We also use a street light format: green, yellow and red for visual aid to make more sense of important information.

Green—Everything is a go!
Stay on track.

Yellow—Use caution.
Be alert because this situation could develop into red. Follow instructions and call parents.

Red— This is an emergency!
Follow instructions carefully and call parents.

Finally, it's important to note that the sitter this book is intended for is an adult or older teenager (at least 16 years of age). We recommend this because of the high responsibility level that is demanded of a child with Type 1 diabetes.

I

What is Type 1 Diabetes?

Type 1 diabetes is a life-altering disease that affects all aspects of daily life. As many as three million Americans, typically children and young adults, are affected. No one has yet discovered the cause, though we do know that it is not a contagious disease and it is not caused by eating too much sugar, or other lifestyle choices.

We all need insulin, which is how blood sugar gets to our cells to be used as energy. During the day our pancreas releases small amounts of insulin. When you start to eat your pancreas releases the insulin for a meal. With Type 1 diabetes, the insulin-producing beta cells in the pancreas die off and the body starves. That is why insulin via shots or a pump needs to be given. For all children with Type 1 diabetes, the dosage of insulin must be accurately calculated according to exercise and the number of carbohydrates eaten.

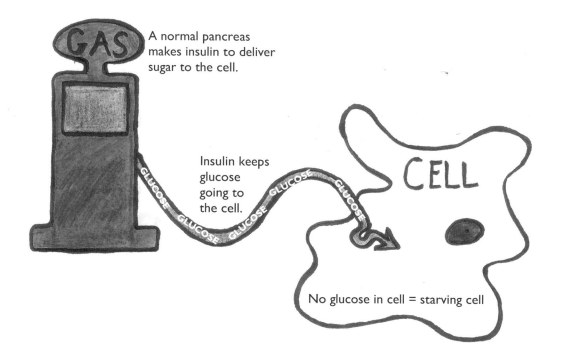

An abnormal pancreas does not make insulin, which means sugar cannot get to the cell.

Common Diabetic Terms

BLOOD SUGAR OR BLOOD GLUCOSE
Comes from the carbohydrates we eat. Our food is digested and then absorbed in the blood stream. Normal blood sugar is 70-100 mg/dl.

BOLUS
A way to correct for a high blood sugar or to cover a snack or meal using an insulin pump. Delivers the "now" insulin. Some pumps have a designated bolus button. You may bolus with partial grams before the meal and then add the rest in during the meal. (Example: meal is a total of 45g of carbs. Bolus 15g before the meal, then 30g during the meal, with food.)

GLUCAGON
Hormone that reverses insulin. It is also in injection form and given as an emergency measure to quickly raise the blood sugar. *For more information, see pages 6-9.*

GLUCOMETER (OR METER)
Device used to test blood sugar requiring a sharp lancet and test strip.

HYPOGLYCEMIA
Low blood sugar. Typically below 70mg/dl. My child's low blood sugar is _____
For more information, see pages 7-8 and 22.

HYPERGLYCEMIA
High blood sugar. Typically above 120mg/dl. My child's high blood sugar starts at _____
For more information, see pages 10-11 and 23.

INSULIN
Hormone required for the body to utilize sugar. There are different types. Long-acting is usually given once to twice a day (also called background insulin). Regular or rapid-acting is usually given with meals. Common names: Lantus®, NovoLog®, Humalog®.

INSULIN PUMP (OR PUMP)
Device, about the size of a deck of cards, that delivers insulin via a small tube inserted in the skin.

KETONES
Byproduct produced when the body is starving and uses protein as energy. Typical in hyperglycemia.

SYRINGE/INSULIN PEN
Device which uses a needle to deliver insulin.

Glucose Meters

Glucometer, glucose meter, meter …. different names for such an important instrument! This little device, about the size of a small cell phone, is used to check the child's blood sugar. This is one of the most critical things the child needs to have with them at all times. It gives a picture of what is going on by measuring current blood sugar levels. Using this information, you will know how to treat the child's blood sugar.

WHEN TO TEST

- Before breakfast
- Before lunch
- Before dinner
- Bedtime
- If you suspect low blood sugar
- During the night if child tends to have low blood sugar while sleeping

WHAT YOU'LL NEED

- Alcohol wipe
- Meter
- Test strip
- Poking device with lancet

WHERE TO TEST

- Fingers, not near fingernail or directly in center of pad, but to the side
- Rotate which fingers are used
- Toes can also be used, particularly for infants.
- Forearm (use clear lancet cap)   Child prefers: _____

HOW TO TEST

- Make sure child washes hands or area to be tested so you get the most accurate reading possible.
- Insert a new lancet into the poking device.
- Insert the test strip into the meter with the sample area facing up and away from the meter. The sample area is where the drop of blood will go. The meter will turn on automatically. If a code number is required, enter the code from the test strip vial so it matches the number on the screen.
- Use the poking device (lancet) to get a drop of blood. Pull back the needle with the lever, place the lancet on testing site, hold firmly, & push the button down to release the needle. A drop of blood should appear.
- If there isn't enough blood, you can hold the hand down to the side of the body to increase blood flow, or gently squeeze the test area.
- When meter indicates "Ready", slide a large drop of blood onto the sample area on test strip.
- Note the blood sugar number on screen. Dispose of the test strip and lancet. _____

Continuous Glucose Monitors (CGMs)

Some kids have a CGM (Continuous Glucose Monitor), which checks their blood sugar 24 hours a day! The child wears a sensor that has a small tube inserted beneath the skin, which transmits the glucose reading every 5 minutes. This does not replace having to manually check blood sugar with a finger stick and a meter. It can, however, alert you to trends of highs or lows so you can keep the child in a normal range. It also can be programmed to set off alarms when the child is low or high, which is especially helpful for kids who can't feel a low, or for heavy sleepers during the night.

If the child wears a CGM, you'll notice that meter readings and sensor readings do not match exactly— this is normal. By manually checking the blood sugar with a finger stick 2-4 times per day, the sensor is calibrated to be more accurate. *(Parents: review how to calibrate.)*

Does the child wear a CGM?   Yes ☐   No ☐   Sometimes ☐

What you need to know about the child's CGM:

_____

_____

_____

_____

_____

What Is Glucagon?

Glucagon is a shot used to reverse insulin in cases of extreme low blood sugars. Glucagon is a hormone just like insulin is, but it raises the blood sugar instead of lowering it. Although glucagon is rarely used, it is critical that you carry this with you at all times in case the child is unconscious or having a seizure from severe low blood sugar.

GLUCAGON KITS ARE LOCATED _____

The red or orange kit comes with a vial of glucagon powder and a fluid-filled syringe. Inject all of the fluid into the vial and gently swirl to mix. You can either use the same large syringe to give the shot, or some parents have a smaller 1.0cc syringe that isn't so intimidating.

While insulin shots are injected into fat, glucagon *can* also be injected into deep muscle, such as front of thigh or the outer arm. Sometimes vomiting can occur with low blood sugar. Keep the child on their side to avoid choking.

HOW TO PREPARE GLUCAGON

1. Take cap off needle.
2. Insert syringe with liquid into vial of powder.
3. Push fluid into vial.
4. Leave syringe in vial.
5. Shake vial until mixed (one uniform solution).
6. Pull back on plunger and draw up all of the fluid into syringe.

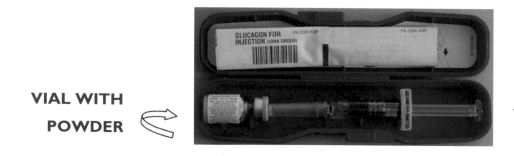

VIAL WITH POWDER ⇦   ⇦ **SYRINGE WITH LIQUID**

What is Low Blood Sugar?

Low blood sugar, or **hypoglycemia**, means there is too little sugar in the blood. The child may feel poorly and you will need to help raise their blood sugar. If not treated right away, the child could become shaky or even lose consciousness. The numbers below indicate where the child should be:

Low _____   Normal _____   High _____

WHAT CAUSES LOW BLOOD SUGAR?

• Too little food • Too much insulin • Strenuous exercise • Illness	• Hot bath _____ _____

SYMPTOMS

Many kids with diabetes know when they are "low", but sometimes a child cannot tell. If you think they are acting out of the ordinary, be safe and check their blood sugar. Treat if needed. It is always better to check!

• Shaky	• Weak	• Drowsy	• Restless sleep,
• Sweaty	• Irritable	• Confused	moaning, nightmares
• Dizzy	• Hungry	• Headache	
• "I feel low."	• "I don't feel good."	• Pale grey or flushed	

WHAT YOU WILL NEED TO TREAT

- Always: Candy with at least 15 grams of carbs, no fat, chocolate or nuts
    - or 3-4 glucose tabs
    - or half a cup of juice (4 oz.)
    - or half a can of regular - not diet - soda (4 oz.)
- Snack with about 15 grams of carbs plus protein, such as crackers and peanut butter, or a granola bar, or a meat and cheese sandwich
- Occasionally: tube of cake gel
- **Rarely: glucagon kit**

WHERE ARE SNACKS AND TREATMENTS LOCATED?

_____

How Do I Treat Low Blood Sugar?

LOW BLOOD SUGAR MUST BE TREATED IMMEDIATELY!

If shaky, dizzy, irritable, sweating or has a headache ...

⬇

Check blood sugar
Low=below 70
Normal=70-120
High=above 200

⬇

If below 70, treat with 15g of carbs such as candy or juice. Wait 15 minutes and retest.

⬇

Repeat treatment of candy/juice at 15 minute intervals until in normal range.

⬇

Finish with a 15g carb snack with **PROTEIN**, such as a granola bar or peanut butter with crackers.

⬇

Call parents. If on pump, stop insulin by suspending pump or removing pump site.

If too shaky to do anything ...

⬇

Help check blood sugar. If this is too difficult, skip this step for now.

⬇

If child cannot chew, squirt a whole tube of cake gel into mouth, then call parents. Wait 15 minutes and retest.

⬇

Repeat treatment of candy/juice at 15 minute intervals until in normal range.

⬇

Finish with a 15g carb snack with **PROTEIN**, such as a granola bar or peanut butter with crackers.

⬇

Call parents. If on pump, stop insulin by suspending pump or removing pump site.

If child is unconscious ...

⬇

Before you call 911, administer _____ units from the glucagon* shot immediately.

⬇

Follow directions in the kit: inject all of the liquid contents into the vial with the powder.

Roll vial between your palms to carefully mix without air bubbles. Pull back _____ units of air.

Inject the air into the vial. Flip the vial with the needle still inside it upside down and pull back _____ units of glucagon.

Inject into the fatty part of the back of arm, thigh or buttocks.

⬇

Call 911. If on pump, stop insulin by suspending pump or removing pump site.

⬇

Roll onto side if vomiting. This could take 10-20 minutes to work. Check blood sugar then.

⬇

Call parents.

---

*See GLUCAGON on next page.

How Do I Give Glucagon?

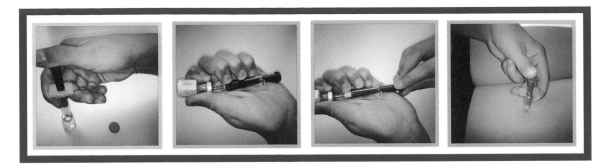

Draw up the amount that corresponds to the child's age below:

    0.3cc (30 units) Children under 6

    0.5cc (50 units) Children 6-18 years

    1.0cc (100 units) Adults over 18 years.

Put needle into the thigh muscle and plunge fluid in. Roll child on his or her side.

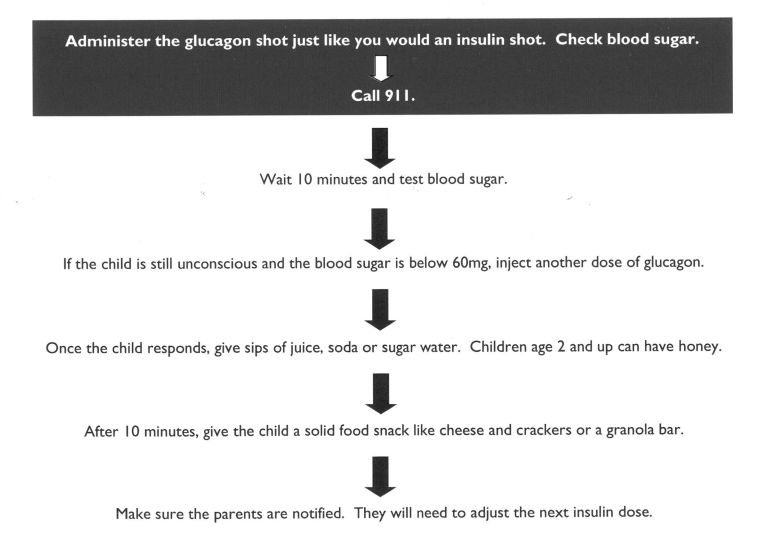

Administer the glucagon shot just like you would an insulin shot. Check blood sugar.

⬇

Call 911.

Wait 10 minutes and test blood sugar.

If the child is still unconscious and the blood sugar is below 60mg, inject another dose of glucagon.

Once the child responds, give sips of juice, soda or sugar water. Children age 2 and up can have honey.

After 10 minutes, give the child a solid food snack like cheese and crackers or a granola bar.

Make sure the parents are notified. They will need to adjust the next insulin dose.

What Is High Blood Sugar?

What is high blood sugar, or **hyperglycemia**? It is an abnormal amount of sugar in the blood with a glucometer reading above 120mg/dl and it needs to be corrected. Causes are: mismatch of food and insulin; not enough insulin; child is growing; infection or illness; emotional stress; excitement. High blood sugar typically does not happen quickly, but rather over a period of time.

My child's blood sugar reading for high blood sugar is above _____

Signs

Very thirsty

Urinating more often

Very hungry

Ketones in urine

Fatigue

Blood sugar reading >150mg/dl

_____

_____

_____

Very high blood sugar symptoms:

Unconscious

Fruity smell

Loss of appetite

Additional Information

An usually high reading could occur if the child didn't wash their hands. The meter could be picking up a trace of juice or sugar. If you suspect this, wash their hands and retest.

_____

How Do I Treat High Blood Sugar?

FOR CHILDREN ON SHOTS

FOR CHILDREN ON PUMPS
Parents, review how your child's pump works.

If blood sugar is over 250 mg/dl

or _____

⬇

Correct via shot with correction of

_____

⬇

Check ketones with next urination or diaper change.

⬇

If moderate or large ketones are present, encourage fluids without sugar, such as water, diet drinks.

⬇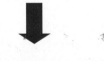

CALL PARENTS

If blood sugar is over 250 mg/dl

or _____

⬇

Correct blood sugar with automatic bolus function.

⬇

Check tubing for cracks or air bubbles. Make sure site is attached, the battery is functioning and that last bolus was given. See page 23 for troubleshooting pumps.

⬇

If blood sugar is above 250 mg/dl two times in a row and there are ketones present, correct with 1 ½ dose. For example, if the pump wants to give 2 units then you would give 2 plus 1 unit to equal 3 units). Site needs to be changed.

_____

_____

_____

⬇

CALL PARENTS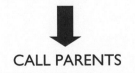

If blood sugar is 150-250 mg/dl, recheck in 2 hours to make sure it is not increasing.

What I Need to Know About Insulin

There are different types of insulins which do different things:

Humalog®, NovoLog® or Apidra®

- Rapid-acting insulin
- Clear liquid
- starts working in 10-15 minutes
- Lasts 3-6 hours

Lantus® or Levemir®

- Long-acting insulin
- Given in a separate syringe
- Starts working in 1-2 hours
- Can last 20-24 hours

NPH®

- Intermediate-acting insulin
- Cloudy, needs to be gently mixed
- Often given in same syringe as a rapid-acting insulin
- Starts working in 1-2 hours
- Lasts up to 15 hours

Remember that the amount or **doses** of these insulins will be **different** and it is extremely important that you know which is which!   It is also critical that you are precise about the dose given. Too much insulin can cause low blood sugar. If this should happen, contact the parents and/or medical provider right away.

Do not inject insulin before a bath or shower because it will be absorbed more quickly, increasing the chance of low blood sugar. If a shower or bath is planned shortly after a meal, give the shot before the meal , then have the child wait about an hour to take the shower or bath.

Rapid ≠ Lantus® (never in same syringe) so ….

Rapid (clear) + NPH® (cloudy) = 1 syringe

Rapid (clear) = 1 separate syringe

+

Lantus® = 1 separate syringe

Parents, consider drawing up insulin prior to short trips out (e.g. movies, dinner, errands). If you will be gone longer, teach the sitter to calculate and draw up insulin according to your correction factors. For more information, see pages 14-15 and Appendix C, D or E pages 40-45.

Injection Sites for Shots and Pumps

FOR KIDS ON SHOTS

The child receives his/her insulin shots: _____

FOR KIDS ON PUMPS

The child inserts his/her infusion site: _____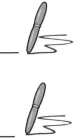

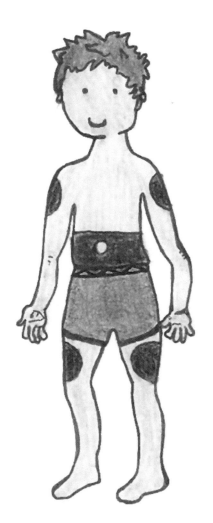 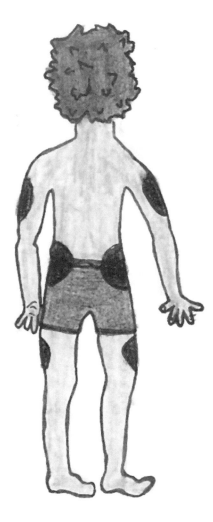

How to Draw Up Insulin
(Rapid-Acting or Lantus®)

Getting Ready

- Gather everything you will need: insulin vial(s), alcohol wipes and a syringe.
- Lay them out on a clean surface on a clean paper towel.
- Wash your hands.
- Vigorously rub tops of the vial(s) with alcohol wipe.

Preparing Shot

For Lantus® insulin alone OR clear (rapid-acting) alone:

First, inject air into insulin vial.

- Using the syringe, pull back the plunger to draw up the amount of air equal to the same dose of Lantus® or rapid insulin. Remove cap.

- With the bottom of bottle on the table, inject all of the air into the vial.

Second, draw up insulin.

- With the needle still in the vial, holding onto both the needle and vial, flip the vial upside down and slowly draw enough insulin beyond the dosage you need.

- While still holding the insulin and syringe together, flick the syringe to float any air bubbles to the top.

- Push excess insulin back into the vial until plunger and dosage line up.

- Pull out the needle.

How to Draw Up Mixed Insulins (Rapid-Acting and NPH®)

PARENTS: CAREFULLY REVIEW AND DEMONSTRATE THE FOLLOWING STEPS!
HAVE SITTER RETURN DEMONSTRATION WITH AN ORANGE.

Getting Ready

- Gather everything you will need: insulin vial(s), alcohol wipes and a syringe.
- Lay them out on a clean surface on a clean paper towel.
- Wash your hands.
- Vigorously rub tops of the vial(s) with alcohol wipe.

Preparing a Mixed Shot

For mixing clear (rapid-acting) and cloudy (NPH®) insulin in one syringe:

First, inject air into insulin vials.

- Mix the vial of cloudy insulin by gently rolling it between your palms to avoid forming bubbles.
- Using the syringe, pull back the plunger to draw up the amount of air equal to the same dose of cloudy insulin.
- With the bottom of bottle on the table, inject all of the air into the cloudy vial. Remove syringe. Set aside.
- Repeat with the clear vial. Do not remove syringe.

Second, draw up insulins.

- Flip the clear insulin vial upside down, leaving **the syringe**. Draw up (pull back) the exact dosage of rapid-acting (clear) insulin you need.
- Now pull out the needle.
- Insert the needle into the cloudy insulin vial, then holding both the vial and syringe, flip upside down.
- Slowly draw back the exact dosage of cloudy insulin needed. (Review dosing on next page.) **Do not to push any insulin back into the vial.**
- Pull out the needle.

Example

- If the dosage is 6 units of cloudy NPH® + 2 units of clear
- Pull back 6 units of air and holding the cloudy vial right-side up, inject the air into the vial. Set aside.
- Pull back 2 units of air and holding the clear vial right-side up, inject the air into that vial.
- Flip the clear vial upside down with the syringe still inside.
- Pull back 2 units of clear insulin. Pull out the syringe.
- With the cloudy vial upside down, insert the syringe and pull back 6 units.
- The total number of units in the syringe should be 6 + 2 = 8 units.

How Do I Give a Shot?

Having to give a shot for the first time can be intimidating. Take a deep breath and relax, remembering that kids will pick up on your confidence. Children with Type 1 diabetes need up to 6 shots of insulin a day, but most will be using the smallest needle possible. You can do this!

- Wash your hands.

- Determine where you are going to give the shot. _____ or _____

- Clean the site with an alcohol wipe and let dry for 10 seconds.

- Lift up the skin with a gentle "pinch". Insulin has to be injected into fat.

- Holding the syringe like a pencil, carefully push the needle all the way into the skin at a 90-degree angle, straight on.

- Slowly push the plunger on the syringe with your index finger.

- Count to three, release your pinch and pull out the needle.

- Dispose of the syringe in a designated container. _____

Practice with an orange. It will help you become familiar with holding the syringe, pressing the plunger, and withdrawing the needle.

Insulin Pens

Some children use insulin pens instead of syringes. Pens are convenient because they come with the insulin already inside. There is a numbered dial that you turn to load the amount of insulin. After that, you just screw on a short needle to the other end. Using pens is just like giving a shot without having to draw up the insulin.

How to give a shot using a pen:

- Set the dial of the pen at zero.

- Prime the pen: after the needle is in place, turn the dial to 2 units while holding pen upright. Push the button to prime, and a drop of insulin will appear on the tip of the needle.

- Next dial up the amount needed for the child. See page 45 (Appendix E) for dosing.

- Determine where you are going to give the shot. _____ or _____

- Clean the site with an alcohol wipe and let dry for 10 seconds.

- Lift up the skin with a gentle "pinch". Insulin has to be injected into fat.

- Holding the insulin pen like a pencil, carefully push the needle all the way through the skin at a 90-degree angle, straight on.

- Slowly push the plunger on the pen.

- Count to 10, release your pinch and pull the pen out.

- Unscrew the needle and dispose of the syringe in a designated container. _____

Common Myths Dispelled

There are many misconceptions and myths about diabetes. Let's set the record straight:

Myth: *Diabetes is contagious.*
Fact: You cannot "catch" diabetes. It is an auto-immune disease that is not contagious.

Myth: *A person with diabetes should eat sugar-free foods.*
Fact: Sugar-free foods, in fact, have a lot of carbohydrates in them. People with diabetes count carbohydrates, not sugar, and sugar-free foods often contain just as many carbs. In fact, one side effect of eating a lot of sugar-free foods is diarrhea, due to the sugar alcohols they contain.

Myth: *Type 1 diabetes is caused by obesity or eating too much sugar.*
Fact: While the risk of getting Type 2 diabetes increases with obesity and a high-sugar diet, the cause of Type 1 diabetes, while as of yet unknown, is thought to be related to genetic factors and the environment.

Myth: *Insulin is the cure for diabetes. Also, people with diabetes can take a pill to control it.*
Fact: Currently, there is not a cure for Type 1 diabetes. Insulin is a hormone that helps a diabetic function as if they had a normal-functioning pancreas. People will Type 2 diabetes can sometimes control their blood sugar levels with a pill.

Myth: *Kids get Type 1 diabetes. Adults get Type 2 diabetes.*
Fact: While Type 1 diabetes used to be called "juvenile diabetes", we now know that people of any age can get Type 1 diabetes. Similarly, the incidence of Type 2 diabetes is increasing in children, especially those with higher risk factors.

Myth: *If a person eats right, exercises and takes their insulin as they should, their blood sugar will be controlled.*
Fact: One of the frustrating aspects of Type 1 diabetes is that controlling blood sugar is a difficult and often discouraging job. Sometimes it's hard to explain or figure out why blood sugar suddenly spikes or drops.

Myth: *People with Type 1 diabetes cannot eat sweets.*
Fact: Like anyone else, moderation of sweets and treats is the key. People with Type 1 diabetes can enjoy sweets like anyone else, as long as they factor in the carbs and have a well-balanced diet.

Myth: *People with Type 1 diabetes should not participate in strenuous activities.*
Fact: People with Type 1 diabetes can do anything anyone else can do, provided they are monitoring their blood sugar and taking care of themselves. Exercise is a wonderful way to keep us all healthy.

Myth: *People with Type 1 diabetes will have long-term complications with eyes, kidneys, hearts, nerves.*
Fact: Controlling blood sugar is the best way to combat long-term complications. A person with Type 1 diabetes will not necessarily have these complications.

Pumps

Insulin pumps are the size of a deck of cards. They are worn all the time, except in water. Because they are not completely waterproof, they need to come off for all water activities, baths and showers. Pumps deliver insulin through a small tube in the body called a cannula. They calculate carbohydrates plus blood sugar readings to decide how much insulin to give.

The child has to eat the amount of food that is given with the pump (or shot). If the child does not want to eat what is served then another option can be given. My child likes _____ for a second option.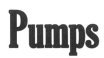

Common Terms

Bolus
A way to correct for a high blood sugar or to cover a snack or meal using an insulin pump. Delivers the "now" insulin. Some pumps have a designated bolus button. You may bolus with partial grams before the meal and then add the rest in during the meal. (Example: meal is a total of 45g of carbs. Bolus 15g before the meal, then 30g during the meal, with food.)

Basal rate
Background insulin. Child receives this all the time. Changes can be made to this per parents.

Temporary Basal
This is an increase or decrease in the percentage of insulin that may be needed for exercise (less) or long car rides (may need more).

Suspend
Stops the basal rate for a set amount of time and then will resume to the normal basal rate. Use for too many lows or when pump needs to be off for a shower.

Parents, please review your child's specific pump with the sitter.
Pump Make & Model

My child's pump is

Make:_____

Model number:_____

Phone number for the manufacturer:_____

Current Pump Settings

There may be a time when you will need to call the doctor or other medical care provider. They will want to know the settings on the child's pump. Do not adjust any pump settings unless explicitly asked by a parent or physician.

Parents, have this completed and updated ahead of time.

Basal settings:

    Max Basal Rate_____

    Standard Basal Rates

    1)_____   _____u/h

    2)_____   _____u/h

    3)_____   _____u/h

    4)_____   _____u/h

    5)_____   _____u/h

    6)_____   _____u/h

Temporary Basal type: ___U/H _____%

Basal Patterns:

    Pattern A/B:

    1)_____/_____   _____/_____u/h

    2)_____/_____   _____/_____u/h

    3)_____/_____   _____/_____u/h

    4)_____/_____   _____/_____u/h

Bolus settings:

    Max Bolus:_____

    Easy Bolus: on/off

    Dual/Square Wave: On/Off

    BG reminders: On/Off

    Bolus wizard set up: On/OFF

    Active insulin time: _____hrs.

Carb Ratios: 1)_____   _____gm/unit

                2)_____   _____gm/unit

                3)_____   _____gm/unit

                4)_____   _____gm/unit

                5)_____   _____gm/unit

                6)_____   _____gm/unit

BG units: _____mg/dl _____mmol/L

Current Pump Settings

Insulin Sensitivity:

1)_____ _____mg/dl/u

2)_____ _____mg/dl/u

3)_____ _____mg/dl/u

4)_____ _____mg/dl/u

Sensor settings

Sensor: On/Off

Glucose alerts: On/Off

Glucose limits: _____-_____mg/dl

High repeat: every _____ hours

Low repeat: every _____ minutes

Cal repeat: ON/Off

Cal reminder: every _____hours

BG units: _____mg/dl **or** _____mmol/L *(check one)*

Transmitter ID number:_____

Weak Signal: On/OFF

BG targets:

1)_____ _____- _____mg/dl

2)_____ _____ -_____ mg/dl

3)_____ _____- _____ mg/dl

4)_____ _____- _____ mg/dl

Utilities

Alarm: Alert Type: _____

Auto Off: On/Off _____hours

Low reservoir: _____units or _____Time

Meter options: On/Off

Meter ID:_____

Remote Options: On/OFF

Remote ID:_____

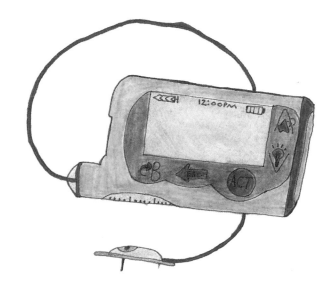

Troubleshooting Pumps: Low Blood Sugar

If you are having problems with low blood sugars **(hypoglycemia)** on an insulin pump, review Problems & Solutions below. If unable to determine the cause, call parents. For causes other than the pump, refer to page 7-8.

Problem	Solution
Too much insulin	• Treat low blood sugar. • Wait 15 minutes, have snack of 15g of carbs. • Closely check carb calculations next time.
Too much exercise	• Sit out of exercise until blood sugar is normal. • Give snack. Types of intense exercise: _____
Not checking blood sugar enough	• Check always before meals and bedtime, as well as 2:00 am. • More frequently if symptoms warrant it.
Two lows in a row	Consider a temporary basal of _____ mg/dl for _____ minutes/hours.

ALWAYS CHECK BLOOD SUGARS BEFORE AND AFTER ACTIVITY

AS WELL AS DURING IF NEEDED.

Exercise uses more blood sugar and creates an opportunity for a low. (For swimming you will need to check blood sugar every two hours, put pump back on and deliver basal rate from last two hours.)

Temporary basal rate of _____% for _____ hour(s) prior to exercise

Temporary basal rate of _____% for _____ hour(s) during exercise

Temporary Basal rate of _____% for _____ hour(s) after exercise

If low twice in a row consider a temporary basal of _____% for _____ hour(s).

Troubleshooting Pumps: High Blood Sugar

If you are having problems with high blood sugars **(hyperglycemia)** on an insulin pump, review Problems & Solutions below. If unable to determine the cause, call parents. For causes other than the pump, refer to page 10-11.

Problem	Solution
High blood sugar over 250 mg/dl: carbohydrate count may have been wrong.	• Correct blood sugar via pump. • Recheck blood sugar in 2 hours.
If blood sugar is over 250 mg/dl again after the first pump correction	• Check the insulin delivery site. ⇒ Make sure there are no air bubbles in the tubing. ⇒ Make sure tubing is connected and pump is delivering insulin. ⇒ Is site securely on? ⇒ Is there any fluid at the site or from the tubing? • Check ketones by peeing on a ketone stick or using wet diaper. If ketones are large, use a 1.5X correction. • Give lots of fluids, especially water. • May need to make a correction injection (per parents) and change insulin site. Call parents at this point.
Insertion site is red, irritated and painful, bloody.	• Change site. • See how much insulin the pump would give to correct the blood sugar, then use this amount to give a manual shot. See page 20 for administering shots.
Failure to deliver insulin per pump.	Give a shot.
Air bubbles in tubing	• Disconnect tubing from body. • Choose fixed bolus from bolus menu and give insulin until bubbles are clear from tubing.
Low battery = No insulin delivery	Change battery. Parents review this.

What to Carry With You & When

Children with Type 1 diabetes cannot leave the house without certain supplies. If the child will be playing outside with friends, riding bikes in the neighborhood, or generally within 10 minutes of home, they should carry a mini kit.

Mini Kit: 5 Minutes From Home

- Glucose meter
- Sugar
- Snack

If the child will be gone for a longer period of time **(for example: going down the street to the park, going to a friend's house, taking a short car ride or going to the pool),** it is up to you to make sure these essentials go with you and the child.

Complete Kit: > 5 Minutes From Home

- Glucagon kit
- Cake gel (with scissors if not a screw-type lid)
- Glucose tabs/candy/juice/or soda
- Follow-up snacks like granola bars
- Syringes (whether on shot therapy and pumps)
- Extra infusion set (for kids on pumps in case site falls off)
- Alcohol wipes
- Insulin if on shot therapy

- Insulin if on pump and more than a 30-minute car ride away
- Insulin pen if on pen therapy
- Batteries _____ type for pumps _____ for meter
- Glucose meter with lancets, poker
- Extra bottle of test strips for meter

Note that insulin should be kept cool (in a lunch bag with an ice pack) and that meters and test strips should never be left in a hot car.

Child's diabetes kit is located: _____

Where Are Supplies Kept?

In case you need to replenish supplies or cannot find something, here is where to look for the following items:

Insulin_____

Syringes_____

Alcohol wipes_____

Lancets_____

Test strips_____

Glucagon kits _____

Cake gel _____

Glucose tabs/candy/juice/or soda_____

Follow-up snacks_____

Infusion sets for pumps_____

Insulin reservoirs for pumps_____

Batteries _____ type for pumps _____ for meters

Meal Time

A child on shot therapy must eat their meals on time. If they are on a carbohydrate counting plan (i.e., a certain amount of carbs must be eaten at a meal), they will need to eat their full meal and snack so it matches their insulin dose. Children on a pump may have more flexibility with the amount of food and the times they eat, but remember that a regular schedule is beneficial to all children — even those who don't have Type 1 diabetes! Good nutrition is important for us all, and while a healthy diet can help control Type 2 diabetes, Type 1 cannot be treated by diet alone. The best diet for all of us, whether we have Type 1 diabetes or not, is healthy foods the majority of the time, along with treats in moderation.

Carbohydrates (Carbs)

The amount of carbs must be accurately calculated because it is the main thing that affects blood sugar. While our bodies automatically release the correct amount of insulin that matches what we eat, as well as when we eat, children with Type 1 diabetes can only get this matching insulin via shot or pump.

For foods that come in a manufacturer's package, you will use the nutrition label to calculate the number of carbs in that particular food. (See page 28 for an example.) Parents may have a nutrition guide for you to use, such as CalorieKing™, or even an app on a SmartPhone or tablet. These tools are very useful for foods without a package, such as fresh meat, vegetables and fruit, or if you are eating out at a restaurant. Most chain and fast-food restaurants have nutritional information available if you ask, or it can be found on their website.

What about those foods that are not packaged? It is very important that you either weigh the food in ounces or grams using a kitchen scale, or use measuring cups and spoons for accuracy. When you have a high-carb food, such as a tablespoon of sugar with 12 g of carbs, you cannot guess at the amount. Otherwise, the amount you use to calculate an insulin dose can cause a child to go high or low.

If a child will be playing at a friend's house, you may need to pack the child's own snack, or find out ahead of time what foods will be there. Check first with the child's parent to make sure an outing like this is okay, and what is the best way to handle other foods.

Meal Time

Children, especially when they are younger, are often not as hungry as they think they are! So if a child <u>thinks</u> they want three slices of pizza, it would be best to serve one slice, see if he or she really does want more, then calculate the insulin dose accordingly. It is ideal to give insulin 15 minutes before a meal but in some instances, you may need to wait.

What do you do if insulin has already been given but the child will not finish their meal? OR if you give too much insulin?   For children on pumps, you can suspend the pump for 30 minutes. Otherwise, see if the child will eat something with enough carbs equal to the extra insulin given. Certain enticing foods, such as honey (for children over 2 years of age) or Nutella®, have high carbs in a spoonful.

While it's tempting to give a treat to the kids you are sitting, it's best to avoid high sugar foods and drinks like juice, soda and candy unless the parent gives you the okay. Even a medium-sized smoothie from your favorite smoothie place can have 70-100 carbs!

There are some different challenges when caring for an infant. It is more likely that you will wait and see what the baby eats before you give insulin. What might you encounter if you are in charge of a baby who eats rice cereal, baby food or formula?   Discuss these things with the parent.

When is it okay for seconds? Typically, for kids on shots, there are no seconds. The amount of insulin has already been dosed to match the food. For kids on pumps, there is more freedom to allow for seconds because you can simply add another dose of insulin for the additional food.

However, there are always exceptions: _____

_____

_____

Parents: on pages 30-31 (Meal Time chart), record the times your child should eat, the insulin dose, and what foods might be prepared.

Sitters: on pages 30-31 (Meal Time chart), record the blood sugars and note any changes to the plan. Give shots 15 minutes before meals, unless there is a chance the child will not eat everything. If this is the case, wait and see how much the child eats, adjust the dosage and give the shot afterwards.

Nutritional Labels

It is important to be able to read a nutrition label so you are correctly calculating the amount of carbs in a food. The biggest factor is **serving size.** If the nutrition label says that 2 tortillas contains 22g total carbs, that is the number you will need to know. If the child eats 1 tortilla, the total carbs is now 11g. You do not need to worry about the number of sugars or fibers at this point.

Nutrition Facts

Serving Size 2 tortillas (51g)
Servings Per Container 6

Amount Per Serving

Calories 110   Calories from Fat 10

	% Daily Value*
Total Fat 1g	2%
Saturated Fat 0g	0%
Trans Fat 0g	
Cholesterol 0mg	0%
Sodium 30mg	1%
Total Carbohydrate 22g	7%
Dietary Fiber 2g	9%
Sugars 0g	
Protein 2g	

Vitamin A 0%	•	Vitamin C 0%
Calcium 2%	•	Iron 4%

*Percent Daily Values are based on a 2,000 calorie diet. Your daily values may be higher or lower depending on your calorie needs:

	Calories:	2,000	2,500
Total Fat	Less than	65g	80g
Saturated Fat	Less than	20g	25g
Cholesterol	Less than	300mg	300mg
Sodium	Less than	2,400mg	2,400mg
Total Carbohydrate		300g	375g
Dietary Fiber		25g	30g

Calories per gram:
Fat 9 • Carbohydrate 4 • Protein 4

Some nutrition labels, such as those for popcorn, rice or pasta, may list the carbs for the food **uncooked**; you will need to have the carbs for the food in its cooked form.

If it is not already portioned out, you will need to weigh or measure the food for accuracy, . Note that proteins such as meat, cheese, nuts and eggs have little or no carbs, if any, unless something has been added such as a sauce or marinade. If a food has less than 5g of carbs, you do not need to give insulin.

The scale is located _____.

Be aware that high fat meals (such as Italian, Chinese, Mexican and fast food) can cause an increase in blood sugar up to 2 hours after being eaten.

Typical Carb Counts

BREAKFAST

Cereal, 1 cup of Cheerios	20g
Milk, 1 cup	12g
Pancake, 4" diameter	11g
Maple syrup, 1 tablespoon	12g
Maple syrup (sugar free), 1/4 cup	7g
Apple, orange, small fresh	15g
Orange juice, 8 oz.	26g
Apple juice, 8 oz.	15g

LUNCH

Strawberries, 1 cup	12g
Grapes, each	1g
Banana, 1/2 of 6"	13g
Bread, regular, one slice	15g
Sandwich, ham & cheese	42g
Peanut butter, 2 tablespoons	7g
Jelly, 2 tablespoons	26g
Yogurt tube	13g
Cheese stick	1g

SNACKS

Chocolate chip cookie	21g
Chips, small bag	15g

DINNER

Chicken nuggets, 5	16g
Pizza, slice, thin crust	10g
Macaroni and cheese, 1 cup	44g

This chart is a tool to record what is going on with the child. It is helpful for you to write all of this out and for the parents to review later. Remember the numbers on this chart are **NOT** a reflection of you as the caretaker of the child. It is just a number. Most of the time it is out of any one person's control.

	Time	Blood Sugar	Insulin Amount
Breakfast			
Snack			
Lunch			
Snack			
Dinner			
Snack			

Insulin Plan

Parents: check which method for insulin administration:

_____15 minutes before meal   _____ ½ before and ½ after meal

_____ with first bite   _____after meal

Notes:_____

Food	Carbs

Developmental Stages

Different kids handle diabetes in different ways. Factors include age, maturity, peers and parenting choices. There is no right or wrong time for a child to handle the responsibilities that come with having Type 1 diabetes. Some kids want to "do it myself" while others may need your help. Here are some guidelines of what to expect from a typical child.

Infants & Toddlers (0-3 years)
- Cannot care for themselves.
- You may have to watch and see how much the child eats, and adjust the dosage of insulin accordingly.

Toddlers & Elementary (3-7 years)
- Need to be supervised by parents or sitter for all diabetic care
- May start to recognize lows at this age
- Should cooperate more than the 0-3 group of children
- Have no concept of time
- Cannot make their own food choices

Elementary (8-12 years)
- Can be taught to check blood sugar
- Learn to draw up and give shots with supervision (age 10-12)
- Learn to count carbs
- Recognize and treat lows
- Can bolus with insulin pump under supervision
- Need general reminders: recheck blood sugars, when to test and treat, can make own food choices
- May remember their own snacks

Junior High & High School (13-18 years)
- Most shots and pump administration
- Can check blood sugar
- Know what foods to eat
- Can count carbs
- Parental guidance is still important: checking on what blood sugar readings are, insulin dosing decisions
- Begin to understand the need for controlled blood sugars

Diabetes Skills

The following list of diabetes skills can be used as a guide to how much supervision is needed. The child can handle the items with a checked box:

☐ Draw up insulin.

☐ Rotate injection sites.

☐ Give own injections.

☐ Make appropriate food choices.

☐ Understand carb to insulin ratio.

☐ Accurately count carbs.

☐ Test blood sugar.

☐ Test for ketones.

☐ Change pump set/site.

☐ Familiar with pump screens and can operate.

☐ Administer own boluses.

☐ Recognize low blood sugar.

☐ Recognize high blood sugar.

☐ Apply correction for high blood sugar (pump).

From Beginning to End

This is an overview of what a typical day looks like. If you ever feel confused, or wonder if you've missed something, it's all right here!

Check blood sugars:
- Before meals
- At bedtime (usually 2 hours after dinner)
- At 2:00 am
- Anytime low or high is suspected
- Remember with a CGM to calibrate blood sugars in the insulin pump.
- If child is wearing a CGM and you suspect a low or high blood sugar, check the insulin pump first rather than with a finger poke and meter.

What do you do with a unusual or unexpected blood sugar?
- Recheck—wash and dry test area with soap and water.
- If blood sugar is still low, then treat (see Low Blood Sugar, pages 7-8, 22).
- If blood sugar is still high, then correct (see High Blood Sugar, pages 10-11, 23).

When do you give insulin?
- For meals and food (see pages 30-31). Count carbohydrates exactly, and weigh and measure food.
- Anytime to correct a high blood sugar (see pages 10-11, 23).

When do I need to recheck a blood sugar?
- 15 minutes after a low (see pages 7-8, 22).
- 2 hours after a high blood sugars. Don't forget to check ketones! (see pages 10-11, 23)

What do I need to go out and about?
- Remember a tester, rapid sugar, snack, extra testing strips (see page 24).

Emergency Contacts

Home address _____

Nearest cross street _____

Home phone _____

Dad's cell _____

Mom's cell _____

Dad's work _____

Mom's work _____

Emergency contact other than parent _____

Endocrinologist (diabetes doctor) _____

Diabetes Care Educator _____

Primary Care Doctor / Pediatrician_____

Location and phone number of where parents will be (restaurant, hotel, friends)

_____

_____

Notes

Notes

Appendix A

Sick Day Management Plan—Shots

Blood sugar is low to normal <150mg Or *_____	Blood sugar is moderate to high 150-300mg Or *_____	Blood sugar is high >300mg Or *_____
Check blood sugar every 1-2 hours. Check urine ketones with each void or diaper change.	Check blood sugar every 2-3 hours. Check urine ketones with each void or diaper change.	Check blood sugar every 2 hours. Check urine ketones with each void or diaper change.
May need to decrease insulin dose: Morning Novolog® by 30-50%. Lantus® may not need adjustment.	May need extra rapid-acting insulin (Novolog® or Humalog®).	May need extra rapid-acting insulin (Novolog® or Humalog®).
For moderate ketones and blood sugar <150, give fluid with sugar (see below). For moderate ketones and blood sugar >150 after sugar fluids are given, go to next column.	For moderate ketones, give Novolog® or Humalog®. 5-10% of total daily dose **or** correction dose x 1.5.	For moderate ketones, give Novolog® or Humalog®. 10% of total daily dose **or** correction dose x 1.5.
Repeat ketone checks every 2 hours until ketones < moderate.	Repeat ketone checks every 2 hours until ketones < moderate.	Repeat ketone checks every 2-3 hours until ketones < moderate.
	For large ketones, give Novolog® or Humalog®. 10-20% of total daily dose **or** correction dose x 1.5. Repeat every 1-2 hours until urine ketones < moderate.	For large ketones, give Novolog® or Humalog®. 20% of total daily dose **or** double correction dose. Repeat every 1-2 hours until urine ketones < moderate.
Give fluids with sugar: Gatorade, apple juice, Pedialyte, popsicles, tea with honey if child is over 1 year of age, or tea with sugar, non-diet soda.	Give fluids: half water, half fluid with sugar, until ketones are negative. Give 1 oz/hour/year of age. Call primary doctor (pediatrician) if infection or fever.	Give water: 1 oz/hour/year of age until blood sugar is <200 mg and ketones are negative. Call primary doctor (pediatrician) if infection or fever.
If vomiting, wait 30-45 minutes, then give only sips of clear fluid every 15 minutes. If vomiting with blood sugar <60mg, you may use a low dose of glucagon, 1 unit per year of age.		

Parents: this should match the ranges you have filled out on page 7.

Appendix B

Sick Day Management Plan—Pumps

Blood sugar is low to normal <150mg Or* _____	Blood sugar is moderate to high 150-300mg Or* _____	Blood sugar is high >300mg Or* _____
Check blood sugar every 1-2 hours. Check urine ketones with each void or diaper change.	Check blood sugar every 2-3 hours. Check urine ketones with each void or diaper change.	Check blood sugar every 2 hours. Check urine ketones with each void or diaper change.
Consider temporary basal rate of 50-75% until blood sugar >80mg. If vomiting and blood sugar is <60mg, disconnect or suspend pump until >80mg.	Give first dose of insulin with a syringe, then change infusion site. May need temp basal rate of 120% if blood sugar remains in the 200's.	Give first dose of insulin with a syringe, then change infusion site. May need temp basal rate of 120% if blood sugar remains in the 200's.
For moderate ketones and blood sugar <150, give fluid with sugar (see below). For moderate ketones and blood sugar >150 after sugar fluids are given, go to next column.	For moderate ketones, give correction dose x 1.5.	For moderate ketones, give correction dose x 1.5.
Repeat ketone checks every 2 hours until ketones < moderate.	Repeat ketone checks every 2 hours until ketones < moderate.	Repeat ketone checks every 2-3 hours until ketones < moderate.
	For large ketones, give correction dose x 2.	For large ketones, give correction dose x 2.
	Repeat every 1-2 hours until urine ketones < moderate.	Repeat every 1-2 hours until urine ketones < moderate.
Give fluids with sugar: Gatorade, apple juice, Pedialyte, popsicles, tea with honey if child is over 1 year of age, or tea with sugar, non-diet soda.	Give fluids: half water, half fluid with sugar, until ketones are negative. Give 1 oz/hour/year of age. Call primary doctor (pediatrician) if infection or fever.	Give water: 1 oz/hour/year of age until blood sugar is <200 mg and ketones are negative. Call primary doctor (pediatrician) if infection or fever.
If vomiting, wait 30-45 minutes, then give only sips of clear fluid every 15 minutes. If vomiting with blood sugar <60mg, you may use a low dose of glucagon, 1 unit per year of age.		

*Parents: this should match the ranges you have filled out on page 7.

39

Appendix C
Sample Injection Schedule For a Day— 2 Shots

Parents: Change according to your child's needs. Fill out factors ahead of time.

Snacks	Because the child on shot or pen therapy is on a regimented meal plan, if he or she is hungry in between meals give a snack less than 10 g carbs, or a protein snack such as cheese, meat, 1/4 cup nuts, protein drink, etc.	

Breakfast
 	
Mixed shot of NOVOLOG® or other rapid-acting insulin
+
NPH long-acting insulin
	1. Check blood sugar. *Target is 70-150 or _____.*
	    BLOOD GLUCOSE = _____
	
	2. The dose of NPH is a fixed amount of _____ units.
	
	CALCULATE DOSE OF RAPID-ACTING INSULIN:
	
	3. FOOD FACTOR
	    Calculate how much insulin is needed for food eaten.
	    Total amount of carbs *divided by* _____ carbs per unit = amount of insulin
	        CARBS _____ ÷ _____ carb ratio = _____
	    Example: 60g carbs ÷ 32 = 1.875 units (Food Factor)
	
	4. CORRECTION FACTOR
	    Calculate how much insulin is needed if blood sugar is above target.
	  • Give 1 unit of insulin per 100 points of glucose above target of 150.
	  • If below 150, there is no need to correct so the factor is 0.
	  • If over 150: subtract 150 from blood glucose and divide by 100.
	  • Blood glucose _____ - 150 ÷ 100 = _____
	  • **Example: if 287 is blood glucose, 287 – 150 = 137**
	  • **137 ÷ 100 = 1.37 units (Correction Factor)**
	
	5. Add FOOD FACTOR to CORRECTION FACTOR
	  • _____ + _____ = _____ total units of insulin
	  • Round up or down to nearest .5 unit
	  • **Example: 1.875 units + 1.37 units = 3.25 units**
	  • **Round up to >>> 3.5 units of NovoLog® if toward the higher end of range, 3 units if toward the lower end.**
		NPH FIXED DOSE
		_____
		
		FOOD FACTOR
		_____
		
		+ CORRECTION FACTOR
		+ _____
		
		= RAPID ACTING INSULIN DOSE
		= _____

Lunch **No Shot**	Check blood sugar. *Target is 70-150 or _____.* BLOOD GLUCOSE = _____	

Appendix C

Sample Injection Schedule For a Day— 2 Shots

Dinner
 	
Mixed shot of NOVOLOG® or other rapid-acting insulin
+
NPH long-acting insulin
	1. Check blood sugar. *Target is 70-150 or* _____.
	     BLOOD GLUCOSE = _____
	
	2. The dose of NPH is a fixed amount of _____ units.
	
	CALCULATE DOSE OF RAPID-ACTING INSULIN:
	
	3. FOOD FACTOR
	     Calculate how much insulin is needed for food eaten.
	     Total amount of carbs *divided by* _____ carbs per unit = amount of insulin
	          CARBS _____ ÷ _____ carb ratio = _____
	     Example: 60g carbs ÷ 32 = 1.875 units (Food Factor)
	
	4. CORRECTION FACTOR
	     Calculate how much insulin is needed if blood sugar is above target.
	• Give 1 unit of insulin per 100 points of glucose above target of 150.
	• If below 150, there is no need to correct so the factor is 0.
	• If over 150: subtract 150 from blood glucose and divide by 100.
	• Blood glucose _____ - 150 ÷ 100 = _____
	• **Example: if 287 is blood glucose, 287 – 150 = 137**
	• **137÷ 100 = 1.37 units (Correction Factor)**
	
	5. Add FOOD FACTOR to CORRECTION FACTOR
	• _____ + _____ = _____ total units of insulin
	• Round up or down to nearest .5 unit
	• **Example: 1.875 units + 1.37 units = 3.25 units**
	• **Round up to >>> 3.5 units of NovoLog® if toward the higher end of range, 3 units if toward the lower end.**
		NPH FIXED DOSE
		
		_____
		
		FOOD FACTOR
		
		_____
		
		+ CORRECTION FACTOR
		+ _____
		
		= RAPID ACTING INSULIN DOSE
		= _____

Bedtime **No Shot**	Check blood sugar. *Target is 70-150 or* _____. BLOOD GLUCOSE = _____ If hungry and blood glucose is in target range, give snack as noted above. If blood glucose is below 100, give a bigger snack, like ice cream, to avoid the danger of going low in the middle of the night.	
Emergencies	"I don't feel good." "I feel shaky." "I have a headache." • Test blood sugar. • If above 250, treat for hyperglycemia (high blood sugar). See pages 10-11. • If above 100 in range, child is okay. He/she can have _____ for headaches. Have child drink water. • If 80-100, child is okay and can have a little snack (small apple, 15g carb granola bar). • If below 70, treat for hypoglycemia (low blood sugar). See pages 7-8. • If below 70 and unconscious, administer glucagon immediately. See pages 8-9.	

Appendix D
Sample Injection Schedule For a Day—3 Shots

Parents: Change according to your child's needs. Fill out factors ahead of time.

Snacks	Because the child on shot or pen therapy is on a regimented meal plan, if he or she is hungry in between meals give a snack less than 10 g carbs, or a protein snack such as cheese, meat, 1/4 cup nuts, protein drink, etc.

| Breakfast

Mixed shot of NOVOLOG® or other rapid-acting insulin
+
NPH long-acting insulin

OR

Separate shots of NOVOLOG® or other rapid-acting insulin
+
Lantus® long-acting insulin | 1. Check blood sugar. *Target is 70-150 or _____.*
    BLOOD GLUCOSE = _____

2. The dose of NPH or Lantus® is a fixed amount of _____ units.

CALCULATE DOSE OF RAPID-ACTING INSULIN:

3. FOOD FACTOR
    Calculate how much insulin is needed for food eaten.
    Total amount of carbs *divided by* _____ *carbs per unit* = amount of insulin
        CARBS _____ ÷ _____ *carb ratio* = _____
    Example: 60g carbs ÷ 32 = 1.875 units (Food Factor)

4. CORRECTION FACTOR
    Calculate how much insulin is needed if blood sugar is above target.
• Give 1 unit of insulin per 100 points of glucose above target of 150.
• If below 150, there is no need to correct so the factor is 0.
• If over 150: subtract 150 from blood glucose and divide by 100.
• Blood glucose _____ - 150 ÷ 100 = _____
• **Example: if 287 is blood glucose, 287 – 150 = 137**
• **137÷ 100 = 1.37 units (Correction Factor)**

5. Add FOOD FACTOR to CORRECTION FACTOR
• _____ + _____ = _____ total units of insulin
• Round up or down to nearest .5 unit
• **Example: 1.875 units + 1.37 units = 3.25 units**
• **Round up to >>> 3.5 units of NovoLog® if toward the higher end of range, 3 units if toward the lower end.** | NPH or Lantus®
FIXED DOSE
_____

FOOD FACTOR
_____

+ CORRECTION FACTOR
+ _____

= RAPID ACTING INSULIN DOSE
= _____ |

| Lunch
No Shot | Check blood sugar. *Target is 70-150 or _____.*
BLOOD GLUCOSE = _____ | |

Appendix D
Sample Injection Schedule For a Day— 3 Shots

Dinner
 	
NOVOLOG®
or other rapid-
acting insulin
	1. Check blood sugar. *Target is 70-150 or* _____.
	   BLOOD GLUCOSE = _____
	
	CALCULATE DOSE OF RAPID-ACTING INSULIN:
	
	2. FOOD FACTOR
	   Calculate how much insulin is needed for food eaten.
	   Total amount of carbs *divided by* _____ *carbs per unit* = amount of insulin
	   CARBS _____ ÷ _____ *carb ratio* = _____
	
	3. CORRECTION FACTOR
	   Calculate how much insulin is needed if blood sugar is above target.
	• Give 1 unit of insulin per 100 points of glucose above target of 150.
	• If below 150, there is no need to correct so the factor is 0.
	• If over 150: subtract 150 from blood glucose and divide by 100.
	• Blood glucose _____ - 150 ÷ 100 = _____
	
	4. Add FOOD FACTOR to CORRECTION FACTOR
	• _____ + _____ = _____ total units of insulin
	• Round up or down to nearest .5 unit
		FOOD FACTOR
		_____
		
		+ CORRECTION
		FACTOR
		+ _____
		
		= RAPID ACTING
		  INSULIN DOSE
		= _____

Bedtime **NPH or** **LANTUS®** **or other long-** **acting insulin**	Check blood sugar. *Target is 70-150 or* _____. BLOOD GLUCOSE = _____ The dose of Lantus® or NPH is a fixed amount of _____ units. *Give shot of* _____ *units of Lantus® or NPH.* If hungry and blood glucose is in target range, give snack as noted above. If blood glucose is below 100, give a bigger snack, like ice cream, to avoid the danger of going low in the middle of the night.	
Emergencies	"I don't feel good." "I feel shaky." "I have a headache." • Test blood sugar. • If above 250, treat for hyperglycemia (high blood sugar). See pages 10-11. • If above 100 in range, child is okay. He/she can have _____ for headaches. Have child drink water. • If 80-100, child is okay and can have a little snack (small apple, 15g carb granola bar). • If below 70, treat for hypoglycemia (low blood sugar). See pages 7-8. • If below 70 and unconscious, administer glucagon immediately. See pages 8-9.	

Appendix E

Sample Injection Schedule For a Day— 4 Shots (Pens)

Snacks	Because the child on shot or pen therapy is on a regimented meal plan, if he or she is hungry in between meals give a snack less than 10 g carbs, or a protein snack such as cheese, meat, 1/4 cup nuts, protein drink, etc.	

Breakfast
 	
NOVOLOG® **(blue pen) or other rapid-acting insulin**
	1. Check blood sugar. *Target is 70-150 or _____.*
	    BLOOD GLUCOSE = _____
	
	CALCULATE DOSE OF RAPID-ACTING INSULIN:
	
	2. FOOD FACTOR
	    Calculate how much insulin is needed for food eaten.
	    Total amount of carbs *divided by* _____ *carbs per unit* = amount of insulin
	         CARBS _____ ÷ _____ *carb ratio* = _____
	    Example: 60g carbs ÷ 32 = 1.875 units (Food Factor)
	
	3. CORRECTION FACTOR
	    Calculate how much insulin is needed if blood sugar is above target.
	• Give 1 unit of insulin per 100 points of glucose above target of 150.
	• If below 150, there is no need to correct so the factor is 0.
	• If over 150: subtract 150 from blood glucose and divide by 100.
	• Blood glucose _____ - 150 ÷ 100 = _____
	• **Example: if 287 is blood glucose, 287 – 150 = 137**
	• **137÷ 100 = 1.37 units (Correction Factor)**
	
	4. Add FOOD FACTOR to CORRECTION FACTOR
	• _____ + _____ = _____ total units of insulin
	• Round up or down to nearest .5 unit
	• **Example: 1.875 units + 1.37 units = 3.25 units**
	• **Round up to >>> 3.5 units of NovoLog® if toward the higher end of range, 3 units if toward the lower end.**
		FOOD FACTOR
		_____
		
		+ CORRECTION FACTOR
		+ _____
		
		= INSULIN DOSE
		= _____

Lunch
 	
NOVOLOG® **(blue pen) or other rapid-acting insulin**
	1. Check blood sugar. *Target is 70-150 or _____.*
	    BLOOD GLUCOSE = _____
	
	CALCULATE DOSE OF RAPID-ACTING INSULIN:
	
	2. FOOD FACTOR
	    Calculate how much insulin is needed for food eaten.
	    Total amount of carbs *divided by* _____ *carbs per unit* = amount of insulin
	         CARBS _____ ÷ _____ *carb ratio* = _____
	
	3. CORRECTION FACTOR
	    Calculate how much insulin is needed if blood sugar is above target.
	• Give 1 unit of insulin per 100 points of glucose above target of 150.
	• If below 150, there is no need to correct so the factor is 0.
	• If over 150: subtract 150 from blood glucose and divide by 100.
	• Blood glucose _____ - 150 ÷ 100 = _____
	
	4. Add FOOD FACTOR to CORRECTION FACTOR
	• _____ + _____ = _____ total units of insulin
	• Round up or down to nearest .5 unit
		FOOD FACTOR
		_____
		
		+ CORRECTION FACTOR
		+ _____
		
		= INSULIN DOSE =
		_____

Appendix E
Sample Injection Schedule For a Day—4 Shots (Pens)

Lunch
 	
NOVOLOG® (blue pen) or other rapid-acting insulin
	1. Check blood sugar. *Target is 70-150 or _____.*
	   BLOOD GLUCOSE = _____
	
	CALCULATE DOSE OF RAPID-ACTING INSULIN:
	
	2. FOOD FACTOR
	   Calculate how much insulin is needed for food eaten.
	   Total amount of carbs *divided by* _____ *carbs per unit* = amount of insulin
	   CARBS _____ ÷ _____ *carb ratio* = _____
	
	3. CORRECTION FACTOR
	   Calculate how much insulin is needed if blood sugar is above target.
	   • Give 1 unit of insulin per 100 points of glucose above target of 150.
	   • If below 150, there is no need to correct so the factor is 0.
	   • If over 150: subtract 150 from blood glucose and divide by 100.
	   • Blood glucose _____ - 150 ÷ 100 = _____
	
	4. Add FOOD FACTOR to CORRECTION FACTOR
	   • _____ + _____ = _____ total units of insulin
	   • Round up or down to nearest .5 unit
		FOOD FACTOR
		_____
		
		+ CORRECTION FACTOR
		+ _____
		
		= INSULIN DOSE
		= _____

Bedtime **LANTUS®** (purple pen) or other long-acting insulin	Check blood sugar. *Target is 70-150 or _____.* BLOOD GLUCOSE = _____ The dose of Lantus® is a fixed amount of _____ units. *Give shot of _____ units of Lantus® (purple pen).* If hungry and blood glucose is in target range, give snack as noted above. If blood glucose is below 100, give a bigger snack, like ice cream, to avoid the danger of going low in the middle of the night.	
Emergencies	"I don't feel good." "I feel shaky." "I have a headache." • Test blood sugar. • If above 250, treat for hyperglycemia (high blood sugar). See pages 10-11. • If above 100 in range, child is okay. He/she can have _____ for headaches. Have child drink water. • If 80-100, child is okay and can have a little snack (small apple, 15g carb granola bar). • If below 70, treat for hypoglycemia (low blood sugar). See pages 7-8. • If below 70 and unconscious, administer glucagon immediately. See pages 8-9.	
Pens	Child washes his/her hands. Wipe injection site and top of pen with alcohol wipe. Dial correct amount of insulin.	

Introduction to Pull-Out Pages For Babysitters

The following pages make up a pull-out section for the babysitter. We recommend placing these important pages by the phone or on the fridge. It's also a great idea to have the whole book nearby.

Allow plenty of time to review the sections with the adult in charge. Make sure the adult is very comfortable with the information they are getting. Remember that they don't have the training you do and may need some time to adjust to your child's medical needs.

DINNER AND A MOVIE

The first section is for the babysitter or adult who is caring for your child while you are out for a few hours. Have the sitter come over first to review your child's needs. Then go over the section and anything that needs to be taught ahead of time (such as giving a shot if it is needed). Learning something new does not always happen overnight. You may want to try out the sitter first while you take a quick trip to the store or some other short outing, then progress to your "dinner and a movie" span of time. The goal is to keep your child safe AND have your sitter be comfortable.

SLEEPOVERS

The first step towards letting your child have a sleepover is establishing a good relationship with the other parents, grandparents or adult in charge. Make sure the adult is comfortable with shots, managing pumps, counting carbohydrates and emergencies. This helps everything become smoother for your child with little stress on the child himself. Before an actual sleepover, we suggest (1) starting with a play date that is not during meal time, then (2) a play date during a meal, and finally (3) the sleepover itself. It may take multiple times to teach the other adult until you find a level of comfort where you can leave your child with this person Several visits also help to not overload the other person with too much information, thus ensuring a successful sleepover!

Again, these sections are for you to tear out and are pages we feel are the absolute essentials for a sleepover. Additionally, you may feel that the following pages are important for your child's safety:

- How to Draw Up Insulin (pages 14-15)
- Appendix C, D or E: Sample Injection Schedule for a Day (pages 40-45) depending on your child

Pull-Out Pages for Babysitters: Dinner and a Movie

This short section of the book, the very basic pages a sitter will need, are ideal for guiding you through the few hours you will be in charge of a child with Type 1 diabetes. Whether the parent runs to the grocery store, goes out for coffee, or is gone for an evening out, this section has you covered. You may not use or need every page, but it is important that you are comfortable with the instructions and that you review them thoroughly with the parent ahead of time. Ask the parents any questions you have before watching the child. And when in doubt, when you are in charge, it is always best to call the parents if you're not sure about something! If you cannot get a hold of the parent then call the endocrinologist—the child's doctor for diabetes. Throughout the book, important information is highlighted in green, yellow or red:

Green—Everything is a go!
Stay on track.

Yellow—Use caution.
Be alert because this situation could develop into red. Follow instructions and call parents.

Red— This is an emergency!
Follow instructions carefully and call parents.

How Do I Treat Low Blood Sugar?

LOW BLOOD SUGAR MUST BE TREATED IMMEDIATELY!

If shaky, dizzy, irritable, sweating or has a headache ...

⬇

Check blood sugar
Low=below 70
Normal=70-120
High=above 200

⬇

If below 70, treat with 15g of carbs such as candy or juice. Wait 15 minutes and retest.

⬇

Repeat treatment of candy/juice at 15 minute intervals until in normal range.

⬇

Finish with a 15g carb snack with PROTEIN, such as a granola bar or peanut butter with crackers.

⬇

Call parents. If on pump, stop insulin by suspending pump or removing pump site.

If too shaky to do anything ...

⬇

Help check blood sugar. If this is too difficult, skip this step for now.

⬇

If child cannot chew, squirt a whole tube of cake gel into mouth, then call parents. Wait 15 minutes and retest.

⬇

Repeat treatment of candy/juice at 15 minute intervals until in normal range.

⬇

Finish with a 15g carb snack with PROTEIN, such as a granola bar or peanut butter with crackers.

⬇

Call parents. If on pump, stop insulin by suspending pump or removing pump site.

If child is unconscious ...

⬇

Before you call 911, administer ____ units from the glucagon* shot immediately.

⬇

Follow directions in the kit: inject all of the liquid contents into the vial with the powder.

Roll vial between your palms to carefully mix without air bubbles. Pull back ____ units of air.

Inject the air into the vial. Flip the vial with the needle still inside it upside down and pull back ____ units of glucagon.

Inject into the fatty part of the back of arm, thigh or buttocks.

⬇

Call 911. If on pump, stop insulin by suspending pump or removing pump site.

⬇

Roll onto side if vomiting. This could take 10-20 minutes to work. Check blood sugar then.

⬇

Call parents.

---

*See GLUCAGON on next page.

How Do I Give Glucagon?

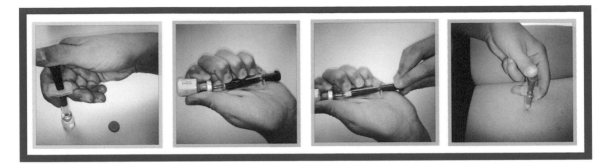

Draw up the amount that corresponds to the child's age below:

0.3cc (30 units) Children under 6 ☐

0.5cc (50 units) Children 6-18 years ☐

1.0cc (100 units) Adults over 18 years. ☐

Put needle into the thigh muscle and plunge fluid in. Roll child on his or her side.

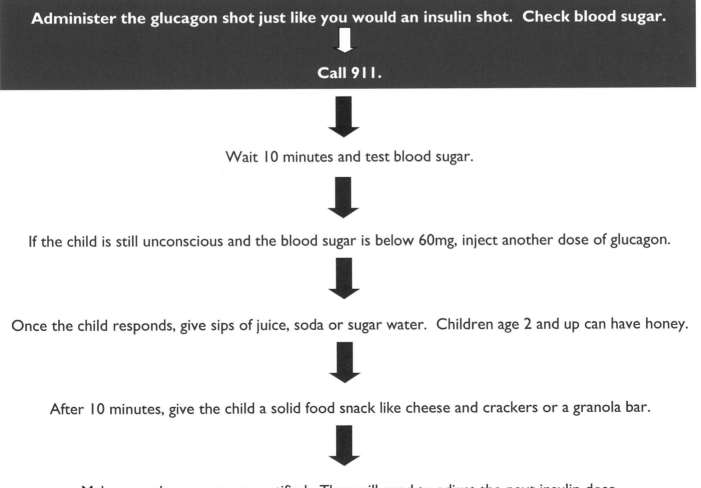

Administer the glucagon shot just like you would an insulin shot. Check blood sugar.

⬇

Call 911.

⬇

Wait 10 minutes and test blood sugar.

⬇

If the child is still unconscious and the blood sugar is below 60mg, inject another dose of glucagon.

⬇

Once the child responds, give sips of juice, soda or sugar water. Children age 2 and up can have honey.

⬇

After 10 minutes, give the child a solid food snack like cheese and crackers or a granola bar.

⬇

Make sure the parents are notified. They will need to adjust the next insulin dose.

Troubleshooting Pumps: Low Blood Sugar

If you are having problems with low blood sugars **(hypoglycemia)** on an insulin pump, review Problems & Solutions below. If unable to determine the cause, call parents.

Problem	Solution
Too much insulin	• Treat low blood sugar. • Wait 15 minutes, have snack of 15g of carbs. • Closely check carb calculations next time.
Too much exercise	• Sit out of exercise until blood sugar is normal. • Give snack. Types of intense exercise: _____
Not checking blood sugar enough	• Check always before meals and bedtime, as well as 2:00 am. • More frequently if symptoms warrant it.
Two lows in a row	Consider a temporary basal of _____ mg/dl for _____ minutes/hours.

ALWAYS CHECK BLOOD SUGARS BEFORE AND AFTER ACTIVITY

AS WELL AS DURING IF NEEDED.

Exercise uses more blood sugar and creates an opportunity for a low. (For swimming you will need to check blood sugar every two hours, put pump back on and deliver basal rate from last two hours.)

Temporary basal rate of _____% for _____ hour(s) prior to exercise

Temporary basal rate of _____% for _____ hour(s) during exercise

Temporary Basal rate of _____% for _____ hour(s) after exercise

If low twice in a row consider a temporary basal of _____% for _____ hour(s).

How Do I Treat High Blood Sugar?

FOR CHILDREN ON SHOTS

If blood sugar is over 250 mg/dl

or _____

⬇

Correct via shot with correction of

_____

⬇

Check ketones with next urination or diaper change.

⬇

If moderate or large ketones are present, encourage fluids without sugar, such as water, diet drinks.

⬇

CALL PARENTS

FOR CHILDREN ON PUMPS
Parents, review how your child's pump works.

If blood sugar is over 250 mg/dl

or _____

⬇

Correct blood sugar with automatic bolus function.

⬇

Check tubing for cracks or air bubbles. Make sure site is attached, the battery is functioning and that last bolus was given. See page 23 in main manual for troubleshooting pumps.

⬇

If blood sugar is above 250 mg/dl two times in a row and there are ketones present, correct with 1 ½ dose. For example, if the pump wants to give 2 units then you would give 2 plus 1 unit to equal 3 units). Site needs to be changed.

_____

_____

_____

⬇

CALL PARENTS

If blood sugar is 150-250 mg/dl, recheck in 2 hours to make sure it is not increasing.

How Do I Give a Shot?

Having to give a shot for the first time can be intimidating. Take a deep breath and relax, remembering that kids will pick up on your confidence. Children with Type 1 diabetes need up to 6 shots of insulin a day, but most will be using the smallest needle possible. You can do this!

- Wash your hands.

- Determine where you are going to give the shot. _____ or _____

- Clean the site with an alcohol wipe and let dry for 10 seconds.

- Lift up the skin with a gentle "pinch". Insulin has to be injected into fat.

- Holding the syringe like a pencil, carefully push the needle all the way into the skin at a 90-degree angle, straight on.

- Slowly push the plunger on the syringe with your index finger.

- Count to three, release your pinch and pull out the needle.

- Dispose of the syringe in a designated container. _____

Practice with an orange. It will help you become familiar with holding the syringe, pressing the plunger, and withdrawing the needle.

Insulin Pens

Some children use insulin pens instead of syringes. Pens are convenient because they come with the insulin already inside. There is a numbered dial that you turn to load the amount of insulin. After that, you just screw on a short needle to the other end. Using pens is just like giving a shot without having to draw up the insulin.

How to give a shot using a pen:

- Set the dial of the pen at zero.

- Prime the pen: after the needle is in place, turn the dial to 2 units while holding pen upright. Push the button to prime, and a drop of insulin will appear on the tip of the needle.

- Next dial up the amount needed for the child. See page 45 (Appendix E) for dosing.

- Determine where you are going to give the shot. _____ or _____

- Clean the site with an alcohol wipe and let dry for 10 seconds.

- Lift up the skin with a gentle "pinch". Insulin has to be injected into fat.

- Holding the insulin pen like a pencil, carefully push the needle all the way through the skin at a 90-degree angle, straight on.

- Slowly push the plunger on the pen.

- Count to 10, release your pinch and pull the pen out.

- Unscrew the needle and dispose of the syringe in a designated container. _____

This chart is a tool to record what is going on with the child. It is helpful for you to write all of this out and for the parents to review later. Remember the numbers on this chart are **NOT** a reflection of you as the caretaker of the child. It is just a number. Most of the time it is out of any one person's control.

	Time	Blood Sugar	Insulin Amount
Breakfast			
Snack			
Lunch			
Snack			
Dinner			
Snack			

Insulin Plan

Parents: check which method for insulin administration:

_____15 minutes before meal   _____ ½ before and ½ after meal

_____ with first bite   _____after meal

Notes:_____

Food	Carbs

Emergency Contacts

Home address _____

Nearest cross street _____

Home phone _____

Dad's cell _____

Mom's cell _____

Dad's work _____

Mom's work _____

Emergency contact other than parent _____

Endocrinologist (diabetes doctor) _____

Diabetes Care Educator _____

Primary Care Doctor / Pediatrician_____

Location and phone number of where parents will be (restaurant, hotel, friends)

_____

_____

Notes

Pull-Out Pages for Babysitters: Sleepovers

Being in charge of a child with Type 1 diabetes can at times feel very overwhelming. Don't worry! The parents of the child went through the exact same thing! These pages are designed to help increase your comfort level with the child. With training and time you will be more comfortable having this child over. Always remember to start slow when having your child's friend over. Start with small play dates, then progress over time to a sleepover (if that is the intention). If you are unsure about what to do, always call the parents for anything that pertains to the child! With your help, the child with Type 1 will be able to have a "normal" sleepover!

Again this section is for you to tear out. These pages are ones we felt as parents are the absolute essentials for a sleepover. Additionally, you might find it helpful to add the following pages:

- How to Draw Up Insulin (pages 14-15)
- Troubleshooting Pumps: High Blood Sugar (page 23)
- Appendix C, D or E Sample Injection Schedule For a Day (pages 40-45), depending on your child

From Beginning to End

This is an overview of what a typical day looks like. If you ever feel confused, or wonder if you've missed something, it's all right here!

Check blood sugars:

- Before meals
- At bedtime (usually 2 hours after dinner)
- At 2:00 am
- Anytime low or high is suspected
- Remember with a CGM to calibrate blood sugars in the insulin pump.
- If child is wearing a CGM and you suspect a low or high blood sugar, check the insulin pump first rather than with a finger poke and meter.

What do you do with a unusual or unexpected blood sugar?

- Recheck—wash and dry test area with soap and water.
- If blood sugar is still low, then treat (see Low Blood Sugar, pages 61-62 and 64).
- If blood sugar is still high, then correct (see High Blood Sugar, page 65).

When do you give insulin?

- For meals and food (see pages 68-69). Count carbohydrates exactly, and weigh and measure food.
- Anytime to correct a high blood sugar (see page 65).

When do I need to recheck a blood sugar?

- 15 minutes after a low (see pages 61-62).
- 2 hours after a high blood sugars. Don't forget to check ketones! (see page 65)

What do I need to go out and about?

- Remember a tester, rapid sugar, snack, extra testing strips (see page 24 in main manual).

Glucose Meters

Glucometer, glucose meter, meter …. different names for such an important instrument! This little device, about the size of a small cell phone, is used to check the child's blood sugar. This is one of the most critical things the child needs to have with them at all times. It gives a picture of what is going on by measuring current blood sugar levels. Using this information, you will know how to treat the child's blood sugar.

WHEN TO TEST

- Before breakfast
- Before lunch
- Before dinner
- Bedtime
- If you suspect low blood sugar
- During the night if child tends to have low blood sugar while sleeping

WHAT YOU'LL NEED

- Alcohol wipe
- Meter
- Test strip
- Poking device with lancet

WHERE TO TEST

- Fingers, not near fingernail or directly in center of pad, but to the side
- Rotate which fingers are used
- Toes can also be used, particularly for infants.
- Forearm (use clear lancet cap)   Child prefers: _____

HOW TO TEST

- Make sure child washes hands or area to be tested so you get the most accurate reading possible.

- Insert a new lancet into the poking device.

- Insert the test strip into the meter with the sample area facing up and away from the meter. The sample area is where the drop of blood will go. The meter will turn on automatically. If a code number is required, enter the code from the test strip vial so it matches the number on the screen.

- Use the poking device (lancet) to get a drop of blood. Pull back the needle with the lever, place the lancet on testing site, hold firmly, & push the button down to release the needle. A drop of blood should appear.

- If there isn't enough blood, you can hold the hand down to the side of the body to increase blood flow, or gently squeeze the test area.

- When meter indicates "Ready", slide a large drop of blood onto the sample area on test strip.

- Note the blood sugar number on screen. Dispose of the test strip and lancet. _____

What is Low Blood Sugar?

Low blood sugar, or **hypoglycemia**, means there is too little sugar in the blood. The child may feel poorly and you will need to help raise their blood sugar. If not treated right away, the child could become shaky or even lose consciousness. The numbers below indicate where the child should be:

Low _____   Normal _____   High _____

WHAT CAUSES LOW BLOOD SUGAR?

• Too little food	• Hot bath
• Too much insulin	_____
• Strenuous exercise	_____
• Illness	

SYMPTOMS

Many kids with diabetes know when they are "low", but sometimes a child cannot tell. If you think they are acting out of the ordinary, be safe and check their blood sugar. Treat if needed. It is always better to check!

• Shaky	• Weak	• Drowsy	• Restless sleep, moaning, nightmares
• Sweaty	• Irritable	• Confused	
• Dizzy	• Hungry	• Headache	
• "I feel low."	• "I don't feel good."	• Pale grey or flushed	

WHAT YOU WILL NEED TO TREAT

- Always: Candy with at least 15 grams of carbs, no fat, chocolate or nuts
    - or 3-4 glucose tabs
    - or half a cup of juice (4 oz.)
    - or half a can of regular - not diet - soda (4 oz.)
- Snack with about 15 grams of carbs plus protein, such as crackers and peanut butter, or a granola bar, or a meat and cheese sandwich
- Occasionally: tube of cake gel
- **Rarely: glucagon kit**

WHERE ARE SNACKS AND TREATMENTS LOCATED?

_____

How Do I Treat Low Blood Sugar?

LOW BLOOD SUGAR MUST BE TREATED IMMEDIATELY!

If shaky, dizzy, irritable, sweating or has a headache …

⬇

Check blood sugar
Low=below 70
Normal=70-120
High=above 200

⬇

If below 70, treat with 15g of carbs such as candy or juice. Wait 15 minutes and retest.

⬇

Repeat treatment of candy/juice at 15 minute intervals until in normal range.

⬇

Finish with a 15g carb snack with PROTEIN, such as a granola bar or peanut butter with crackers.

⬇

Call parents. If on pump, stop insulin by suspending pump or removing pump site.

If too shaky to do anything …

⬇

Help check blood sugar. If this is too difficult, skip this step for now.

⬇

If child cannot chew, squirt a whole tube of cake gel into mouth, then call parents. Wait 15 minutes and retest.

⬇

Repeat treatment of candy/juice at 15 minute intervals until in normal range.

⬇

Finish with a 15g carb snack with PROTEIN, such as a granola bar or peanut butter with crackers.

⬇

Call parents. If on pump, stop insulin by suspending pump or removing pump site.

If child is unconscious …

⬇

Before you call 911, administer _____ units from the glucagon* shot immediately.

⬇

Follow directions in the kit: inject all of the liquid contents into the vial with the powder.

Roll vial between your palms to carefully mix without air bubbles. Pull back _____ units of air.

Inject the air into the vial. Flip the vial with the needle still inside it upside down and pull back _____ units of glucagon.

Inject into the fatty part of the back of arm, thigh or buttocks.

⬇

Call 911. If on pump, stop insulin by suspending pump or removing pump site.

⬇

Roll onto side if vomiting. This could take 10-20 minutes to work. Check blood sugar then.

⬇

Call parents.

---

*See GLUCAGON on next page.

How Do I Give Glucagon?

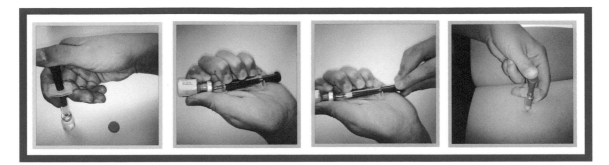

Draw up the amount that corresponds to the child's age below:

    0.3cc (30 units) Children under 6

    0.5cc (50 units) Children 6-18 years

    1.0cc (100 units) Adults over 18 years.

Put needle into the thigh muscle and plunge fluid in. Roll child on his or her side.

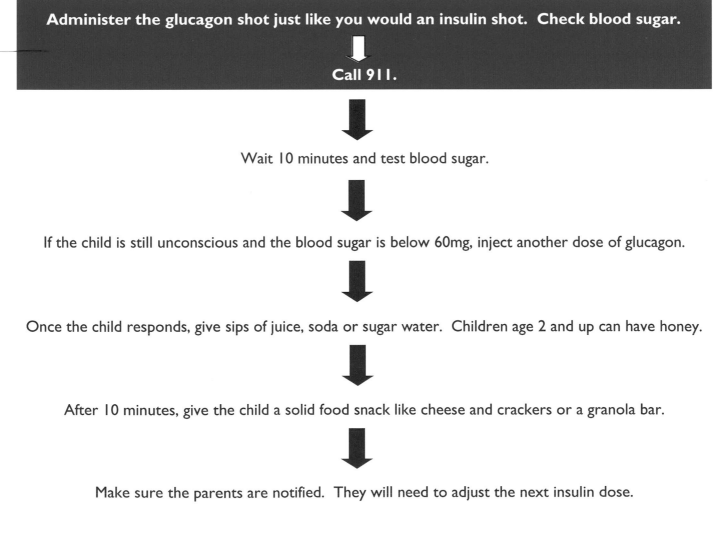

Administer the glucagon shot just like you would an insulin shot. Check blood sugar.

Call 911.

Wait 10 minutes and test blood sugar.

If the child is still unconscious and the blood sugar is below 60mg, inject another dose of glucagon.

Once the child responds, give sips of juice, soda or sugar water. Children age 2 and up can have honey.

After 10 minutes, give the child a solid food snack like cheese and crackers or a granola bar.

Make sure the parents are notified. They will need to adjust the next insulin dose.

Troubleshooting Pumps: Low Blood Sugar

If you are having problems with low blood sugars **(hypoglycemia)** on an insulin pump, review Problems & Solutions below. If unable to determine the cause, call parents. For causes other than the pump, refer to page 61-62.

Problem	Solution
Too much insulin	• Treat low blood sugar. • Wait 15 minutes, have snack of 15g of carbs. • Closely check carb calculations next time.
Too much exercise	• Sit out of exercise until blood sugar is normal. • Give snack. Types of intense exercise: _____
Not checking blood sugar enough	• Check always before meals and bedtime, as well as 2:00 am. • More frequently if symptoms warrant it.
Two lows in a row	Consider a temporary basal of _____ mg/dl for _____ minutes/hours.

ALWAYS CHECK BLOOD SUGARS BEFORE AND AFTER ACTIVITY

AS WELL AS DURING IF NEEDED.

Exercise uses more blood sugar and creates an opportunity for a low. (For swimming you will need to check blood sugar every two hours, put pump back on and deliver basal rate from last two hours.)

Temporary basal rate of _____% for _____ hour(s) prior to exercise

Temporary basal rate of _____% for _____ hour(s) during exercise

Temporary Basal rate of _____% for _____ hour(s) after exercise

If low twice in a row consider a temporary basal of _____% for _____ hour(s).

How Do I Treat High Blood Sugar?

FOR CHILDREN ON SHOTS

If blood sugar is over 250 mg/dl

or _____

⬇

Correct via shot with correction of

_____

⬇

Check ketones with next urination or diaper change.

⬇

If moderate or large ketones are present, encourage fluids without sugar, such as water, diet drinks.

⬇

CALL PARENTS

FOR CHILDREN ON PUMPS
Parents, review how your child's pump works.

If blood sugar is over 250 mg/dl

or _____

⬇

Correct blood sugar with automatic bolus function.

⬇

Check tubing for cracks or air bubbles. Make sure site is attached, the battery is functioning and that last bolus was given. See page 23 in main manual for troubleshooting pumps.

⬇

If blood sugar is above 250 mg/dl two times in a row and there are ketones present, correct with 1 ½ dose. For example, if the pump wants to give 2 units then you would give 2 plus 1 unit to equal 3 units). Site needs to be changed.

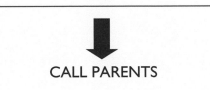

⬇

CALL PARENTS

If blood sugar is 150-250 mg/dl, recheck in 2 hours to make sure it is not increasing.

How Do I Give a Shot?

Having to give a shot for the first time can be intimidating. Take a deep breath and relax, remembering that kids will pick up on your confidence. Children with Type 1 diabetes need up to 6 shots of insulin a day, but most will be using the smallest needle possible. You can do this!

- Wash your hands.

- Determine where you are going to give the shot. _____ or _____

- Clean the site with an alcohol wipe and let dry for 10 seconds.

- Lift up the skin with a gentle "pinch". Insulin has to be injected into fat.

- Holding the syringe like a pencil, carefully push the needle all the way into the skin at a 90-degree angle, straight on.

- Slowly push the plunger on the syringe with your index finger.

- Count to three, release your pinch and pull out the needle.

- Dispose of the syringe in a designated container. _____

Practice with an orange. It will help you become familiar with holding the syringe, pressing the plunger, and withdrawing the needle.

Insulin Pens

Some children use insulin pens instead of syringes. Pens are convenient because they come with the insulin already inside. There is a numbered dial that you turn to load the amount of insulin. After that, you just screw on a short needle to the other end. Using pens is just like giving a shot without having to draw up the insulin.

How to give a shot using a pen:

- Set the dial of the pen at zero.

- Prime the pen: after the needle is in place, turn the dial to 2 units while holding pen upright. Push the button to prime, and a drop of insulin will appear on the tip of the needle.

- Next dial up the amount needed for the child. See page 45 (Appendix E) for dosing.

- Determine where you are going to give the shot. _____ or _____

- Clean the site with an alcohol wipe and let dry for 10 seconds.

- Lift up the skin with a gentle "pinch". Insulin has to be injected into fat.

- Holding the insulin pen like a pencil, carefully push the needle all the way through the skin at a 90-degree angle, straight on.

- Slowly push the plunger on the pen.

- Count to 10, release your pinch and pull the pen out.

- Unscrew the needle and dispose of the syringe in a designated container. _____

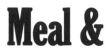Meal &

This chart is a tool to record what is going on with the child. It is helpful for you to write all of this out and for the parents to review later. Remember the numbers on this chart are **NOT** a reflection of you as the caretaker of the child. It is just a number. Most of the time it is out of any one person's control.

	Time	Blood Sugar	Insulin Amount
Breakfast			
Snack			
Lunch			
Snack			
Dinner			
Snack			

Insulin Plan

Parents: check which method for insulin administration:

_____15 minutes before meal   _____ ½ before and ½ after meal

_____ with first bite   _____after meal

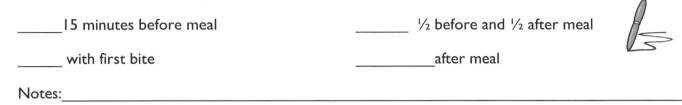

Notes:_____

Food	Carbs

Emergency Contacts

Home address _____

Nearest cross street _____

Home phone _____

Dad's cell _____

Mom's cell _____

Dad's work _____

Mom's work _____

Emergency contact other than parent _____

Endocrinologist (diabetes doctor) _____

Diabetes Care Educator _____

Primary Care Doctor / Pediatrician_____

Location and phone number of where parents will be (restaurant, hotel, friends)

_____

_____

Notes

References

Chase, H. Peter, and David M. Maahs. *Understanding diabetes: a handbook for people who are living with diabetes.* 12th ed. Denver, Colo.: Children's Diabetes Foundation, 2011. Print.

"Developmental Stages and Diabetes." *Colorado Kids With Diabetes.* N.p., n.d. Web. 4 Apr. 2013. <http:www.coloradokidswithdiabetes.org

"Sick Day Management Guidelines for Type 1 Diabetes." *Pediatric Endocrine Associates.* Pediatric Endocrine Associates, n.d. Web. 29 Apr. 2013. <http://denverpedendo.com>.

"Pump Settings" chapter adapted from www.medtronicdiabetes.com/support/download-library/workbooks.

Pen illustration: www.clker.com *(free clipart).*

CPSIA information can be obtained at www.ICGtesting.com
Printed in the USA
BVIW12n0342161216
471003BV00011B/150